<u>Timeless style: A Man's Guide to Classic Dressing.</u>

Table of Contents

Foreword

Acknowledgments

Introduction: Embracing Timeless Style

Chapter 1: Understanding Classic Men's Fashion

- The Evolution of Men's Fashion
- Key Elements of Classic Dressing
- The Importance of Fit and Proportion

Chapter 2: Building a Timeless Wardrobe

- Wardrobe Essentials for Every Man
- Investing in Quality: Fabrics and Construction
- Tailoring: The Foundation of Classic Dressing

Chapter 3: Mastering the Art of Suiting

- The Anatomy of a Well-Tailored Suit
- Choosing the Right Suit for Your Body Type
- Suiting Etiquette: Dressing for Different Occasions

Chapter 4: Dressing for Success: Business Attire

- The Essentials of Business Dressing
- Power Dressing: Projecting Confidence and Authority
- Business Casual: Striking the Right Balance

Chapter 5: Casual Elegance: Weekend and Leisure Wear

- **The Art of Casual Dressing**
- **Weekend Essentials: Smart Casual and Beyond**
- **Dressing for Outdoor Activities: Sportswear and Beyond**

Chapter 6: The Finishing Touches: Accessories and Grooming

- **Elevating Your Look with Accessories**
- **The Gentleman's Guide to Grooming**
- **Maintaining Your Wardrobe: Care and Storage Tips**

Chapter 7: Icons of Style: Drawing Inspiration from the Masters

- **Timeless Style Icons: From Classic Hollywood to Modern-Day Influencers**
- **Lessons in Style: What We Can Learn from the Masters**
- **Creating Your Own Signature Style**

Chapter 8: Navigating Trends: Incorporating Contemporary Fashion

- **Incorporating Trends with Timeless Pieces**
- **The Art of Balance: Mixing Classic and Contemporary Styles**
- **Knowing When to Embrace or Avoid Trends**

Chapter 9: Dressing for Special Occasions

- **Formal Dressing: Black Tie and Beyond**
- **Wedding Attire: Navigating Dress Codes with Elegance**
- **Dressing for Celebrations and Milestones**

Chapter 10: Beyond Fashion: Cultivating Confidence and Presence

- **The Psychology of Dressing Well**
- **Confidence and Self-Expression through Fashion**
- **Embracing Timeless Style as a Lifestyle Choice**

Conclusion: Embracing Your Personal Journey in Timeless Style

Foreword

In a world where fashion trends come and go like passing seasons, there exists a timeless elegance that transcends the whims of fleeting fads. "Timeless Style: A Man's Guide to Classic Dressing" is not just a book; it's a celebration of the enduring allure of classic fashion.

As we navigate through the maze of ever-changing styles, it becomes increasingly evident that true style is not about following the latest trends but about embracing a timeless aesthetic that exudes confidence, sophistication, and authenticity. This book is a testament to the art of dressing well, not just for the moment, but for a lifetime.

In these pages, you'll discover the essential principles of classic dressing, from the impeccable fit of a well-tailored suit to the subtle nuances of accessorising with elegance. Drawing inspiration from the timeless icons of style and the sartorial traditions that have stood the test of time, "Timeless Style" offers practical advice and timeless wisdom for the modern gentleman.

But beyond mere fashion advice, this book is an invitation to cultivate a personal style that reflects who you are and what you stand for. It's about understanding the power of clothing not just as a means of covering the body but as a form of self-expression and a statement of character.

Whether you're a seasoned sartorialist or a novice in the world of menswear, "Timeless Style" is your indispensable guide to mastering the art of classic dressing. So, dive in, explore, and embark on a journey toward sartorial excellence that will not only transform your wardrobe but elevate your entire outlook on life.

Here's to timeless style, enduring elegance, and the pursuit of sartorial perfection.

Warm regards,

Ashlay Homme

<u>**Acknowledgments**</u>

I would like to express my heartfelt gratitude to my family for their unwavering support and encouragement throughout the journey of writing this book. Your love, patience, and belief in me have been my guiding light, and I am deeply grateful for your constant encouragement and inspiration.

To my dear friends Marc, Darren, Michael and Keith, thank you for your unwavering friendship, encouragement, and inspiration. Your camaraderie has been a source of strength and motivation, and I am grateful for the countless conversations and shared moments that have enriched my life.

In the process of writing this book, I have drawn inspiration from the timeless wisdom of Alan Flusser. His seminal work, "Dressing the Man: Mastering the Art of Permanent Fashion," has been a constant source of inspiration and guidance, and I highly recommend it to anyone seeking to delve deeper into the principles of classic dressing.

To all those who have contributed to this journey in ways big and small, thank you for your support, encouragement, and belief in this project. This book would not have been possible without your contributions, and I am truly grateful for your presence in my life.

With deepest gratitude,

Ash

Introduction: Embracing Timeless Style

In a world where trends come and go with the blink of an eye, there exists a realm of fashion that transcends the fleeting whims of passing fads. Some may call it "Traditional" but I prefer to call it "Elemental" because I believe that there are essential elements that make a style timeless.

Today there seems to be a resurgence of classic men's fashion, where the principles of style are as enduring as they are elegant. This in part seems to be driven by the desire for men to identify value in their masculinity and also in part a longing for simpler times. These things are reflected in the art of dressing well, not just for the moment, but for a lifetime.

The Essence of Timeless Style

Timeless style is more than just a fashion statement; it's a way of life. It's about embracing a mindset that values quality over quantity, simplicity over extravagance, and refinement over excess. At its core, timeless style is a celebration of the enduring allure of classic menswear – a symphony of clean lines, understated elegance, and impeccable craftsmanship.

Navigating the Fashion Landscape

In today's fast-paced world, navigating the fashion landscape can be a daunting task. With trends constantly evolving and new styles emerging every season, it's easy to feel overwhelmed and lost in a sea of options. But amidst the chaos, timeless style stands as a beacon of stability and sophistication – a timeless aesthetic that transcends the vagaries of fashion.

The Journey Begins

I am excited to help you embark on this journey through the world of timeless style. Together, we will explore the principles of classic menswear, from the impeccable fit of a well-tailored suit to the subtle nuances of accessorising with elegance. Along the way, we'll draw inspiration from the timeless icons of style and the sartorial traditions that have stood the test of time.

So, whether you're a seasoned sartorialist or a novice in the world of menswear, I hope to help you to embrace the art of masculine style and embark on a journey that will not only transform your wardrobe but elevate your entire outlook on life.

Welcome to the world of timeless style – where elegance is eternal, sophistication is timeless, and authenticity is everything.

Let the journey begin.

Chapter 1: Understanding Classic Men's Fashion

Fashion is a dynamic reflection of culture, society, and individual expression. In the realm of men's fashion, the evolution of style has been a journey through time, influenced by historical events, cultural shifts, and the changing roles of men in society. Understanding the roots and principles of classic men's fashion is essential for mastering the art of timeless dressing.

The Evolution of Men's Fashion

Men's fashion has undergone significant transformations throughout history, shaped by various factors including social norms, technological advancements, and artistic movements. From the opulent attire of ancient civilizations to the tailored suits of the 20th century, the evolution of men's fashion is a rich tapestry of style and innovation.

- Ancient Civilizations: In ancient civilizations such as Egypt, Greece, and Rome, clothing served both practical and symbolic purposes. Garments were crafted from natural fibres such as linen and wool, reflecting the climate and resources of the region. Clothing styles were often draped and tailored to enhance the physique while also conveying social status and identity.

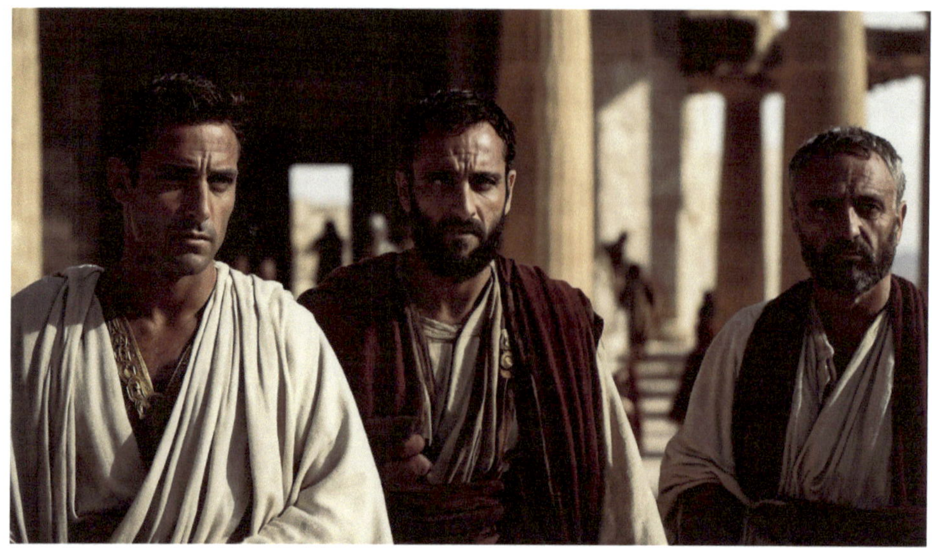

No, I don't expect you to dress like this. Well not unless you are going to a party!

- Middle Ages and Renaissance: The Middle Ages witnessed the emergence of elaborate garments adorned with intricate embroidery and luxurious fabrics. The Renaissance period brought a revival of classical aesthetics, with a focus on proportion, symmetry, and balance in clothing design. Men's fashion during this era was characterised by voluminous sleeves, doublets, and hose, reflecting the opulence of the nobility.
- 18th and 19th Centuries: The 18th century saw the rise of the three-piece suit, consisting of a coat, waistcoat, and breeches, as the standard attire for men of the upper class. With the Industrial Revolution came advancements in textile manufacturing and garment production, leading to the mass production of clothing and the democratisation of fashion. The 19th century witnessed the transition from elaborate court attire to more streamlined and functional clothing, influenced by the rise of the bourgeoisie and the ideals of the Enlightenment.

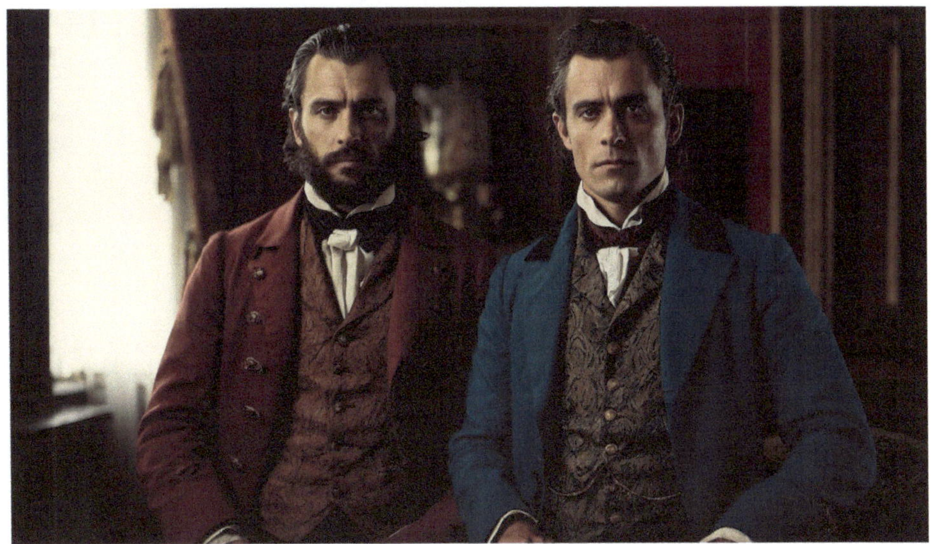

There is a reason that women love period dramas!

- 20th Century and Beyond: The 20th century brought radical changes to men's fashion, driven by technological innovation, cultural shifts, and global events. From the iconic suits of the 1920s jazz age to the casual elegance of 1950s Hollywood, each decade was defined by distinct fashion trends and style icons. The latter half of the 20th century saw the emergence of subcultures such as the hippies, punks, and hip-hop enthusiasts, each leaving their mark on the fashion landscape.

Key Elements of Classic Dressing

Classic dressing is rooted in timeless principles that transcend fleeting trends and fads. At its core, classic dressing is about simplicity, refinement, and elegance. Understanding the key elements of classic dressing is essential for cultivating a wardrobe that stands the test of time.

- Timeless Silhouettes: Classic dressing emphasises clean lines, well-defined silhouettes, and understated elegance. From the tailored silhouette of a well-fitted suit to the effortless drape of a cashmere sweater, timeless silhouettes form the foundation of classic men's fashion.
- Quality Materials: Classic dressing values quality over quantity, prioritising garments crafted from premium materials that age gracefully and withstand the test of time. From fine wool and cashmere to supple leather and sturdy denim, quality materials elevate the look and feel of classic attire.
- Neutral Colours and Versatile Patterns: Classic dressing embraces a neutral colour palette of timeless hues such as navy, charcoal, camel, and olive, complemented by versatile patterns such as stripes, checks, and herringbone. These timeless colours and patterns allow for effortless coordination and timeless sophistication.

The Importance of Fit and Proportion

In the realm of classic dressing, fit and proportion are paramount. A well-tailored garment not only enhances the wearer's physique but also exudes confidence and refinement. Understanding the importance of fit and proportion is essential for mastering the art of classic men's fashion.

- Tailored Fit: Classic dressing favours garments that are tailored to fit the individual's body proportions, creating a streamlined silhouette that flatters the physique. Whether it's the precise fit of a bespoke suit or the tailored silhouette of a dress shirt, attention to fit elevates the overall aesthetic of classic attire.
- Proportionate Silhouettes: Classic dressing emphasises proportionate silhouettes that balance the body's

proportions and create visual harmony. From the proportions of a suit jacket's lapels to the length of trousers and sleeves, achieving balance and proportion is essential for creating a polished and sophisticated look. This is why many opt for a good custom suit over factory made. However, there is nothing to say that a good tailor can't adjust an existing suit to suit your body.

Keep these principles in mind as we continue. They are the backbone of looking and feeling great in your clothing.

Chapter 2: Building a Timeless Wardrobe

In the realm of classic men's fashion, building a timeless wardrobe is akin to laying the foundation of a grand architectural masterpiece. It requires careful consideration, attention to detail, and a deep appreciation for the enduring principles of style. In this chapter, we delve into the essential elements of building a wardrobe that stands the test of time.

Wardrobe Essentials for Every Man

At the heart of every timeless wardrobe lies a collection of essential pieces that form the building blocks of classic dressing. These wardrobe essentials are versatile, timeless, and effortlessly stylish, serving as the backbone of a well-rounded wardrobe.

- The Crisp White Shirt: A timeless classic that exudes sophistication and versatility, the crisp white shirt is a wardrobe staple that can be dressed up or down for any occasion.

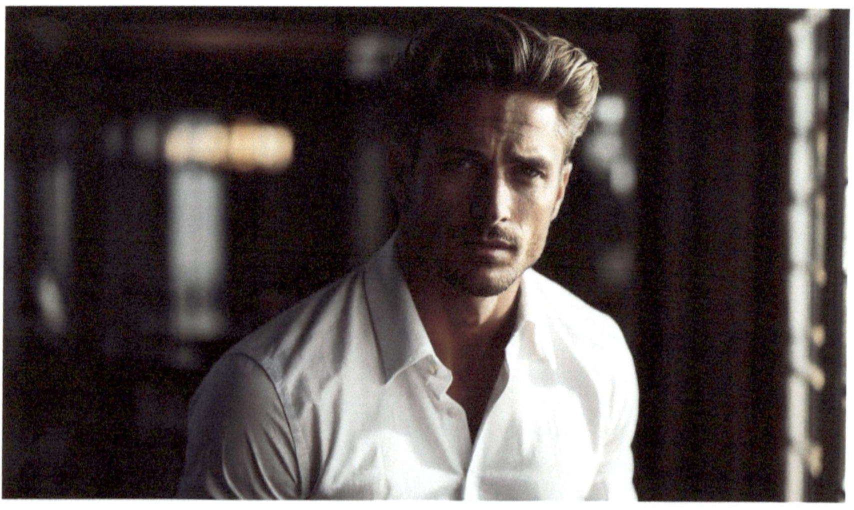

Get a white shirt before working on your smouldering pout!

- The Tailored Suit: A well-tailored suit is the epitome of timeless elegance. Whether it's a classic navy blue suit for formal occasions or a versatile charcoal grey suit for everyday wear, investing in quality tailoring is essential for achieving a polished and sophisticated look.
- The Classic Trench Coat: A timeless outerwear piece that never goes out of style, the classic trench coat is both practical and stylish, making it a must-have for every man's wardrobe.

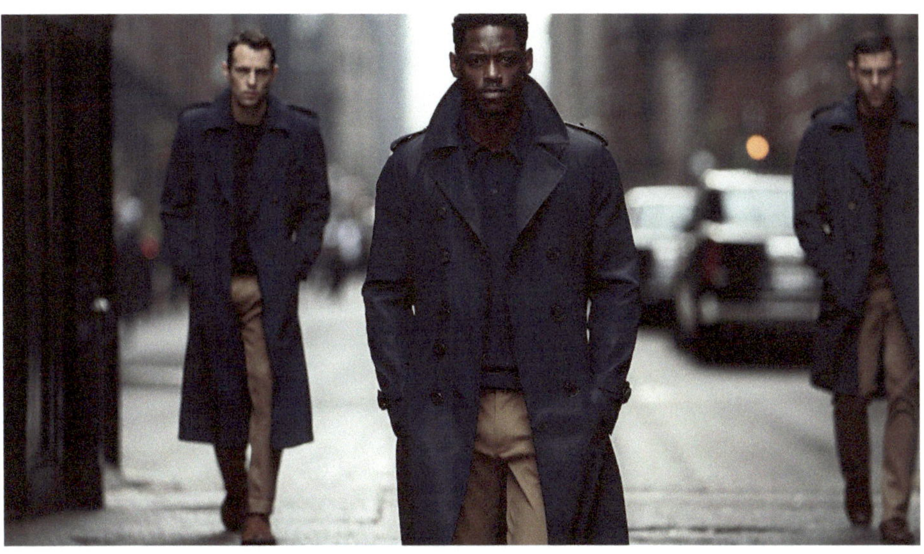

Classic Trench Coat loved by heroes and villains alike!

- The Versatile Knitwear: From the timeless elegance of a fine merino wool sweater to the casual comfort of a classic crewneck sweatshirt, versatile knitwear pieces add texture and dimension to any outfit.
- The Timeless Accessories: A collection of timeless accessories such as a quality leather belt, a classic watch, and a pair of well-crafted leather shoes add the perfect

finishing touch to any ensemble, elevating the overall look with understated elegance.

Investing in Quality: Fabrics and Construction

When it comes to building a timeless wardrobe, quality is paramount. Investing in garments crafted from premium materials and impeccable construction ensures longevity, durability, and timeless elegance.

- Premium Fabrics: From the luxurious softness of cashmere to the durability of fine wool and the timeless elegance of silk, investing in garments crafted from premium fabrics elevates the look and feel of classic attire, ensuring comfort and sophistication with every wear.

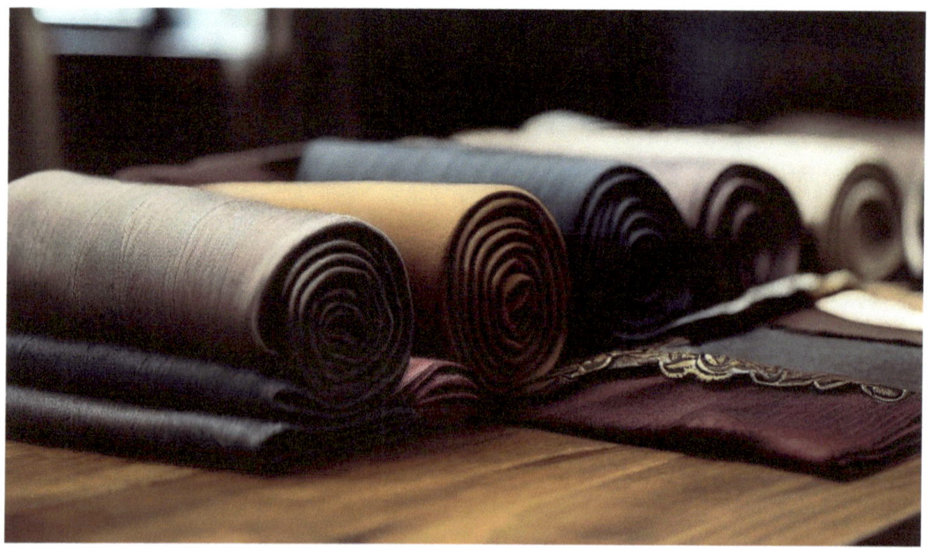

Manners makes the man. Fabric enhances him!

- Impeccable Construction: Attention to detail is key when it comes to timeless dressing. From the precision of hand-stitched seams to the artistry of tailored construction, garments crafted with impeccable construction techniques exude quality, refinement, and timeless elegance.

Tailoring: The Foundation of Classic Dressing

At the heart of classic dressing lies the art of tailoring – the meticulous craft of shaping and refining garments to achieve the perfect fit and silhouette. Tailoring is the foundation of classic dressing, transforming ordinary garments into timeless masterpieces of style and sophistication.

- The Perfect Fit: A well-tailored garment not only enhances the wearer's physique but also exudes confidence and refinement. Whether it's the precise fit of a bespoke suit or the tailored silhouette of a dress shirt, attention to fit is essential for achieving a polished and sophisticated look.
- Customization and Personalisation: Tailoring offers the opportunity for customisation and personalisation, allowing individuals to create garments that reflect their unique style and preferences. From selecting the perfect fabric and design details to achieving the ideal fit and silhouette, the art of tailoring empowers individuals to curate a wardrobe that is truly timeless and personalised.

Building a timeless wardrobe is a journey of craftsmanship, refinement, and personal expression, and with careful consideration and attention to detail, every man can create a wardrobe that stands the test of time.

Chapter 3: Mastering the Art of Suiting

In the realm of classic men's fashion, the tailored suit reigns supreme as the epitome of timeless elegance and sophistication. Mastering the art of suiting requires a deep understanding of the anatomy of a well-tailored suit, the nuances of selecting the right suit for your body type, and the etiquette of dressing for different occasions. In this chapter, we delve into the essential elements of mastering the art of suiting with style and confidence.

The Anatomy of a Well-Tailored Suit

A well-tailored suit is a masterpiece of craftsmanship, precision, and attention to detail. Understanding the anatomy of a well-tailored suit is essential for achieving a polished and sophisticated look that exudes confidence and elegance.

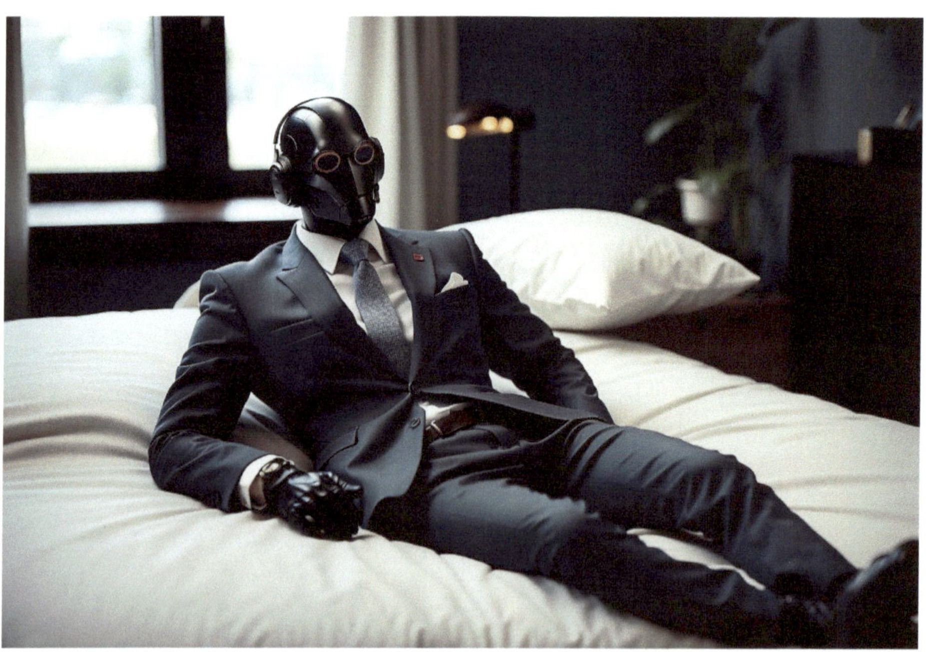

A well tailored suit is Timeless!

- The Jacket: The jacket is the centrepiece of a well-tailored suit, setting the tone for the entire ensemble. Key elements of a well-tailored jacket include a structured shoulder, a defined waist, and a clean, streamlined silhouette. The lapels, buttons, pockets, and vents are carefully crafted to enhance the overall aesthetic and functionality of the jacket.
- The Trousers: The trousers of a well-tailored suit are tailored to perfection, with a flattering fit that complements the wearer's physique. The rise, waistband, and leg width are tailored to achieve a clean, streamlined silhouette, while the length is adjusted to ensure a precise break and elegant drape.
- The Shirt: The shirt worn with a tailored suit should be crisp, clean, and well-fitted, with a collar that frames the face and cuffs that peek out elegantly from the jacket sleeves. The fabric, colour, and pattern of the shirt should complement the suit while adding depth and dimension to the overall ensemble.

Choosing the Right Suit for Your Body Type

When it comes to selecting the right suit for your body type, fit is key. A well-fitted suit not only enhances your physique but also exudes confidence and sophistication. Understanding your body type and selecting suits that flatter your silhouette is essential for mastering the art of suiting with style and confidence.

- Athletic Body Type: For those with an athletic body type characterised by broad shoulders and a narrow waist, opt for suits with structured shoulders and a tapered waist to accentuate your physique. Avoid overly boxy or loose-fitting styles that may obscure your natural proportions.

- Slim Body Type: If you have a slim body type with narrow shoulders and a slender frame, opt for suits with a slim-cut silhouette that follows the natural lines of your body. Avoid oversized or baggy styles that may overwhelm your frame and opt for lightweight fabrics that drape elegantly without adding bulk.
- Full Body Type: For those with a fuller body type characterised by a wider waist and fuller chest, opt for suits with a more relaxed fit that allows for comfortable movement without feeling restrictive. Look for suits with a slightly longer jacket length and trousers with a higher rise to create a balanced silhouette.

Suiting Etiquette: Dressing for Different Occasions

Dressing appropriately for different occasions is an essential aspect of mastering the art of suiting with style and confidence. Whether it's a formal business meeting, a social event, or a special occasion, understanding suiting etiquette and dressing accordingly ensures that you make a lasting impression for all the right reasons.

- Business Attire: When dressing for business, opt for classic, conservative suits in neutral colours such as navy, charcoal grey, or black. Pair your suit with a crisp white shirt, a subtle patterned tie, and polished leather shoes for a professional and polished look.
- Social Events: For social events such as weddings, cocktail parties, or evening receptions, opt for suits in bolder colours or patterns to make a statement. Experiment with different textures, fabrics, and accessories to add personality and

flair to your ensemble while still maintaining a refined and elegant aesthetic.

- Special Occasions: For special occasions such as black-tie events or formal celebrations, opt for a classic tuxedo or dinner jacket in black or midnight blue. Pair your tuxedo with a crisp white shirt, a black bow tie, and polished patent leather shoes for a timeless and sophisticated look that commands attention.

We will go further into this in our next few chapters, but for now be rest assured that with careful consideration and attention to detail, mastering the art of suiting with style and confidence is within reach for every man.

Chapter 4: Dressing for Success: Business Attire

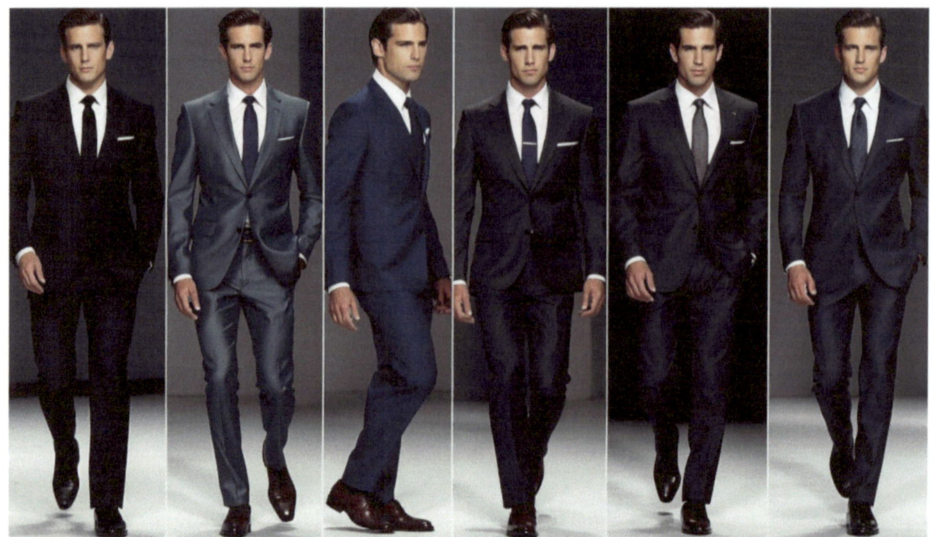

Business suits convey a sense of power and professionalism.

In the corporate world, dressing for success goes beyond mere fashion; it's a powerful tool for projecting confidence, authority, and professionalism. In this chapter, we delve into the essential elements of business attire, the art of power dressing, and the nuances of striking the right balance with business casual attire.

The Essentials of Business Dressing

Business attire sets the tone for professionalism and competence in the workplace. The essentials of business dressing are rooted in classic menswear principles, emphasising clean lines, impeccable tailoring, and attention to detail.

- The Classic Suit: A well-tailored suit in neutral colours such as navy, charcoal grey, or black is the cornerstone of business dressing. Opt for a single-breasted, two-button jacket with structured shoulders and a tailored fit for a polished and professional look.

- The Crisp White Shirt: A crisp, white dress shirt is a timeless essential in business attire. Choose a shirt with a classic spread collar and French cuffs for added sophistication, and ensure a perfect fit that allows for ease of movement without excess fabric.
- The Conservative Tie: A conservative tie in a solid colour or subtle pattern adds a touch of elegance to your business ensemble. Opt for silk ties in classic colours such as navy, burgundy, or dark green, and avoid bold or flashy patterns that may detract from your professional image.
- The Polished Shoes: Polished leather shoes in black or dark brown complete your business ensemble with a touch of refinement. Choose classic oxford or derby shoes with a sleek silhouette and minimal detailing for a timeless and sophisticated look.

Power Dressing: Projecting Confidence and Authority

Power dressing is more than just a fashion statement; it's a strategic tool for projecting confidence, authority, and leadership in the workplace. The art of power dressing lies in choosing garments and accessories that command attention and convey a sense of professionalism and competence.

- Tailored Silhouettes: Power dressing emphasises tailored silhouettes that accentuate your physique and convey a sense of confidence and authority. Opt for suits with structured shoulders, a defined waist, and a clean, streamlined silhouette that exudes sophistication and professionalism.
- Bold Colours and Patterns: Incorporating some colours and patterns into your business attire can add personality and

flair while still maintaining a professional aesthetic. Just don't overdo it! Experiment with subtle patterns such as pinstripes or window panes, or add a pop of colour with a statement tie or pocket square.

- Attention to Detail: Attention to detail is key in power dressing, from the precise fit of your suit to the subtle nuances of your accessories. Ensure that your garments are well-tailored and properly pressed, and pay attention to the finer details such as cufflinks, tie bars, and pocket squares for a polished and professional look.

Business Casual: Striking the Right Balance

Business casual attire strikes a delicate balance between professionalism and comfort, offering a more relaxed alternative to traditional business attire while still maintaining a polished and professional appearance.

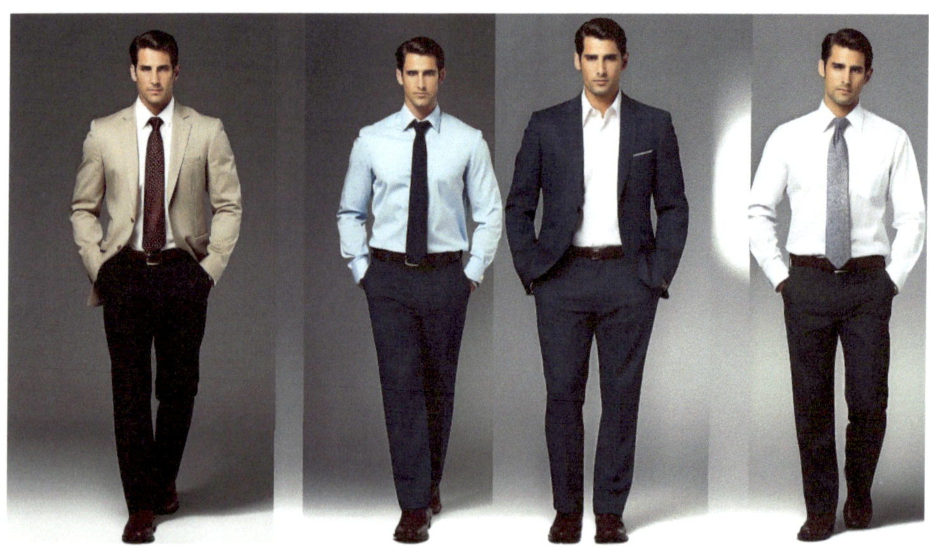

Business casual allows you to mix and match and find your own style

- Smart Separates: Business casual attire often consists of smart separates such as tailored trousers, dress shirts, and blazers in coordinating colours and fabrics. Opt for well-fitted garments with clean lines and minimal embellishments for a sophisticated and professional look.
- Casual Accessories: Business casual attire allows for more casual accessories such as leather belts, loafers, and chukka boots. Choose accessories that complement your outfit while still maintaining a professional aesthetic, and avoid overly casual or flashy items that may detract from your overall appearance.
- Dressing for the Occasion: When dressing in business casual attire, it's important to consider the specific requirements of the occasion. Whether it's a client meeting, a networking event, or a casual Friday in the office, choose attire that is appropriate for the setting while still reflecting your personal style and professionalism.

By mastering the principles of business attire, you can project confidence, authority, and professionalism in the workplace while still expressing your personal style and individuality.

Chapter 5: Casual Elegance: Weekend and Leisure Wear

In the realm of men's fashion, casual elegance is a delicate balance of comfort, style, and sophistication. As we step away from the confines of the workplace, weekend and leisure wear offer an opportunity to express personal style while embracing a relaxed and effortless aesthetic. In this chapter, we explore the art of casual dressing, the essentials of smart casual attire, and the nuances of dressing for outdoor activities with style and elegance.

The Art of Casual Dressing

Casual dressing is an art form that combines comfort with style, creating effortlessly chic ensembles that exude confidence and individuality. The key to mastering the art of casual dressing lies in selecting versatile pieces that can be mixed and matched to create a variety of stylish looks.

- Casual Tops: From classic crewneck t-shirts to casual button-down shirts, casual tops form the foundation of casual dressing. Choose tops in quality fabrics and classic colours such as white, navy, or grey for a timeless and versatile wardrobe.
- Relaxed Bottoms: Relaxed bottoms such as chinos, jeans, and shorts are essential for creating casual yet stylish ensembles. Opt for well-fitted bottoms in neutral colours and classic cuts that flatter your physique while offering comfort and ease of movement.
- Layering: Layering is key to achieving a stylish and versatile casual look. Experiment with layering lightweight sweaters, cardigans, and jackets over casual tops for added warmth and dimension, while still maintaining a relaxed and effortless aesthetic.

Weekend Essentials: Smart Casual and Beyond

Smart casual attire strikes the perfect balance between casual comfort and refined elegance, offering a versatile and stylish option for weekend wear and leisure activities. From casual outings to social events, mastering the essentials of smart casual attire ensures that you look polished and put-together while still embracing a relaxed and effortless aesthetic.

- The Polo Shirt: The polo shirt is a timeless essential in smart casual attire, offering a stylish and versatile option for weekend wear. Choose polo shirts in quality fabrics and classic colours such as navy, black, or white, and pair them with chinos or tailored shorts for a classic and refined look.

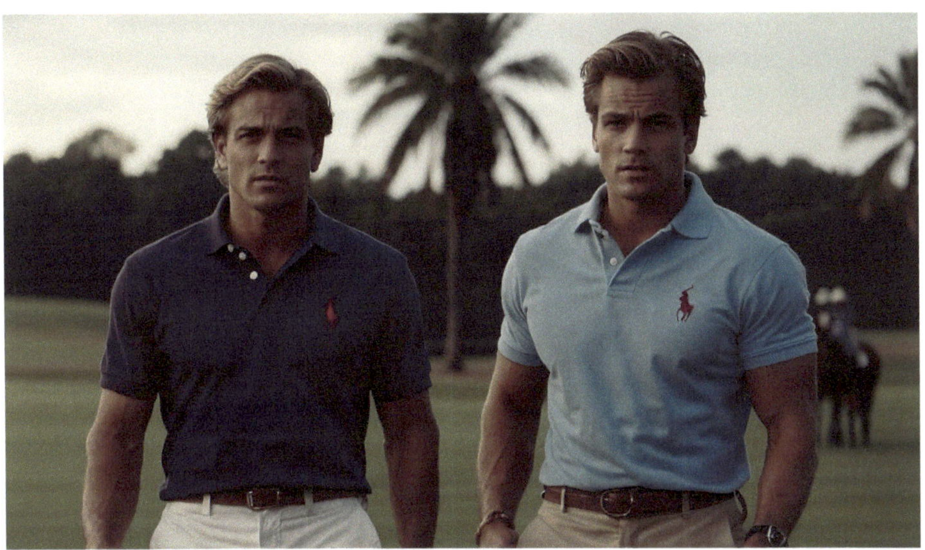

Polo Bros!

- The Casual Blazer: A casual blazer is a versatile wardrobe staple that adds polish and sophistication to any outfit. Opt for unstructured blazers in lightweight fabrics such as linen or cotton for a relaxed and effortless aesthetic, and pair them with casual tops and bottoms for a stylish and refined look.

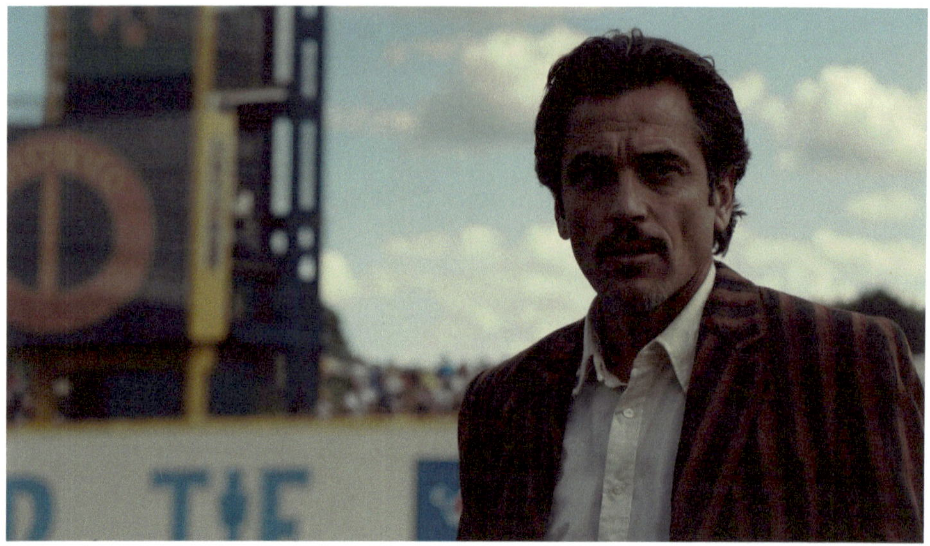

Casual Blazers really allow you to experiment with colour and style.

- The Casual Shoe: Casual shoes such as loafers, boat shoes, and sneakers are essential for completing your smart casual ensemble. Choose shoes in classic styles and neutral colours that complement your outfit while still offering comfort and versatility for all-day wear.

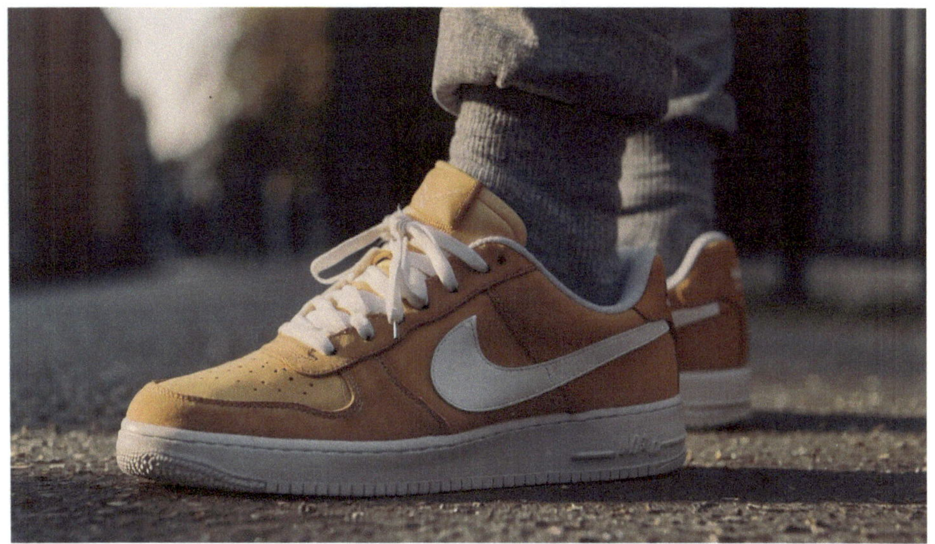

Need I say more!

Dressing for Outdoor Activities: Sportswear and Beyond

Dressing for outdoor activities requires a balance of style, functionality, and comfort, ensuring that you look and feel your best while engaging in leisure pursuits. Whether it's a weekend hike, a round of golf, or a casual game of tennis, mastering the essentials of outdoor sportswear ensures that you stay stylish and comfortable in any setting.

- Performance Fabrics: Performance fabrics such as moisture-wicking materials, breathable mesh, and stretchy elastane are essential for outdoor sportswear, offering comfort and functionality for all-day wear. Opt for garments crafted from performance fabrics that offer moisture management, UV protection, and temperature regulation for maximum comfort and performance.
- Functional Accessories: Functional accessories such as baseball caps, sunglasses, and performance socks are essential for outdoor activities, offering protection from the

elements while still maintaining a stylish and sporty aesthetic. Choose accessories in durable materials and classic designs that complement your outdoor ensemble while offering functionality and comfort.

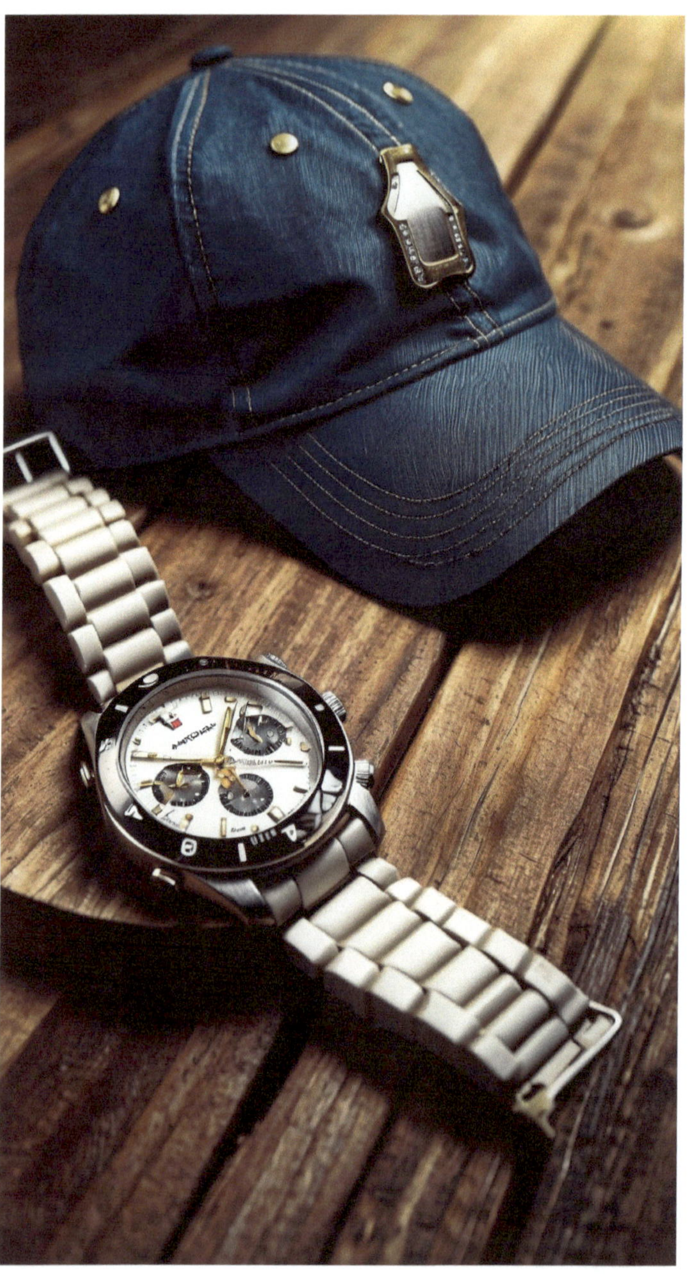

- Versatile Outerwear: Versatile outerwear such as lightweight jackets, windbreakers, and waterproof coats are essential for outdoor activities, offering protection from the elements while still maintaining a stylish and sporty aesthetic. Opt for outerwear in classic styles and neutral colours that complement your outdoor ensemble while offering functionality and versatility for all-weather wear.

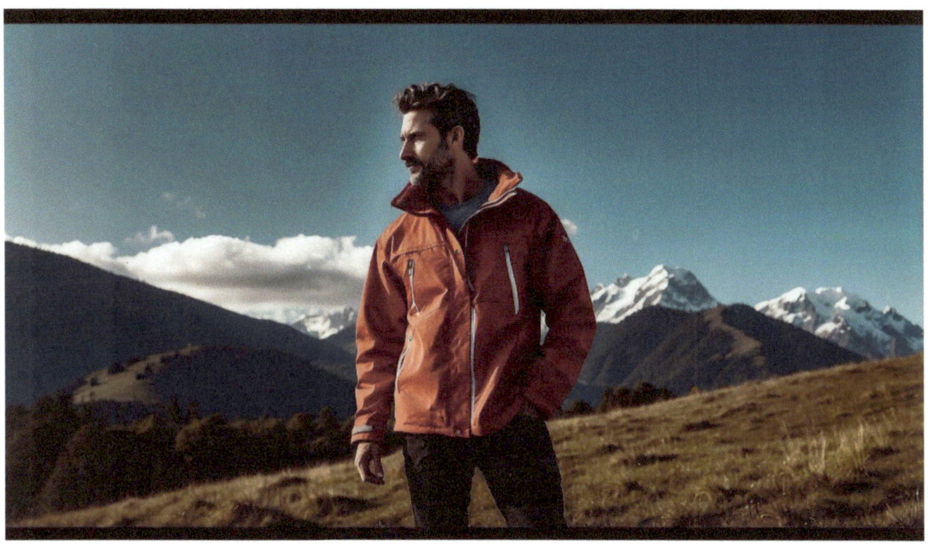

Just because nobody is around, does not mean that you can't be stylish!

By mastering the principles of casual elegance, you can embrace a relaxed and effortless aesthetic while still looking polished and put-together for weekend wear and leisure activities.

Chapter 6: Dressing for Special Occasions

Special occasions call for attire that goes beyond the everyday, reflecting the significance and solemnity of the event while still exuding style and elegance. In this chapter, we explore the nuances of dressing for special occasions, from formal events to weddings and celebrations, with grace and sophistication.

Formal Dressing: Black Tie and Beyond

Formal dressing is the epitome of elegance and sophistication, requiring attire that is refined, polished, and appropriate for the occasion. From black tie events to gala dinners and opera performances, mastering the art of formal dressing ensures that you make a lasting impression for all the right reasons.

- Black Tie Attire: Black tie attire is the pinnacle of formal dressing, requiring a tuxedo or dinner jacket in black or midnight blue paired with a crisp white dress shirt, a black bow tie, and polished leather shoes. Opt for classic accessories such as cufflinks, a pocket square, and a dress watch to complete your black tie ensemble with style and sophistication.
- White Tie Attire: White tie attire is reserved for the most formal of occasions, requiring a tailcoat or evening coat in black or midnight blue paired with a white dress shirt generally with a wing collar, black or midnight blue trousers which, may also have a satin stripe, a white bow tie, and black patent leather shoes. Accessories such as a top hat, white gloves, and formal jewellery add a touch of regal elegance to your white tie ensemble, ensuring that you stand out for all the right reasons.

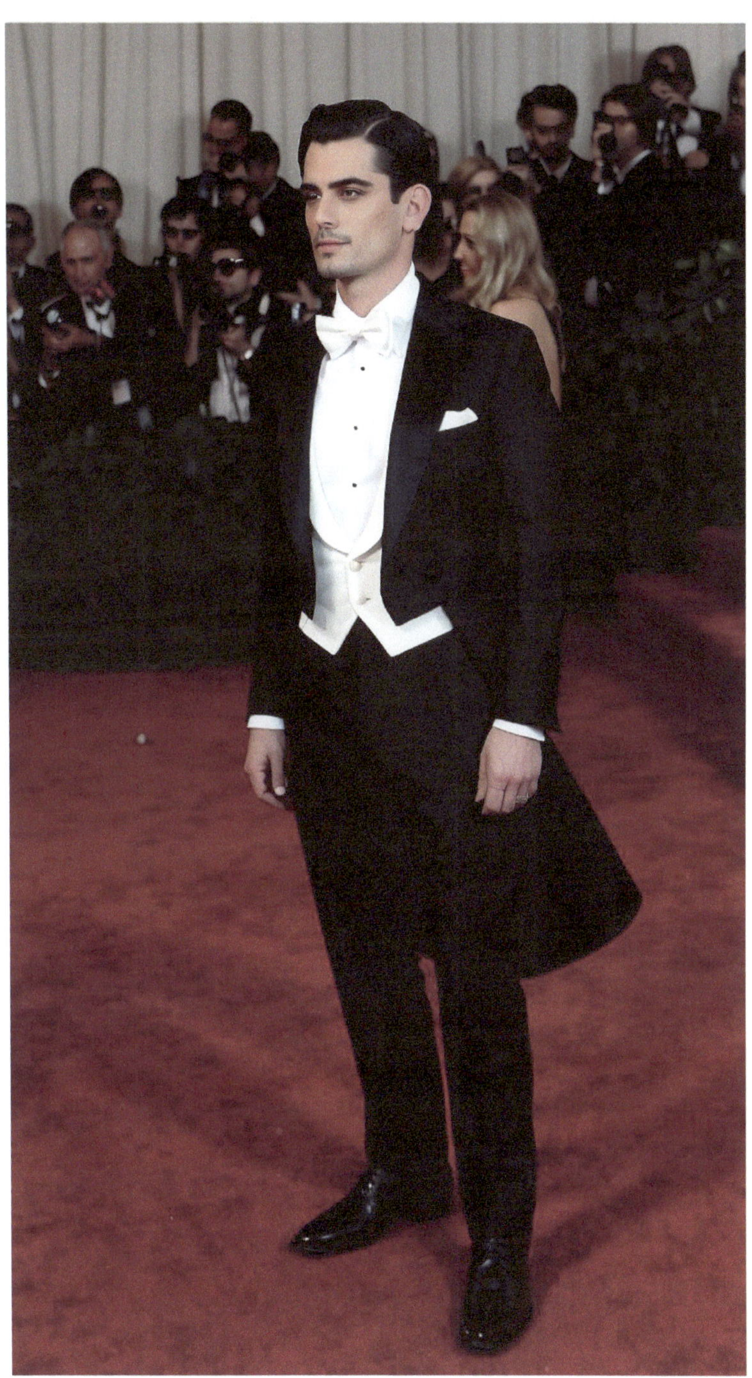

Classic white tie for when you hit the red carpet

Wedding Attire: Navigating Dress Codes with Elegance

Weddings are a celebration of love and commitment, requiring attire that is elegant, tasteful, and respectful of the occasion. Navigating wedding dress codes with grace and elegance ensures that you look and feel your best while honouring the significance of the event.

- Formal Wedding Attire: For formal weddings, opt for classic and timeless attire such as a tailored suit in charcoal grey or navy paired with a crisp white dress shirt, a patterned tie, and polished leather shoes. Pay attention to the specific dress code outlined on the wedding invitation, and choose attire that reflects the formality and elegance of the occasion.

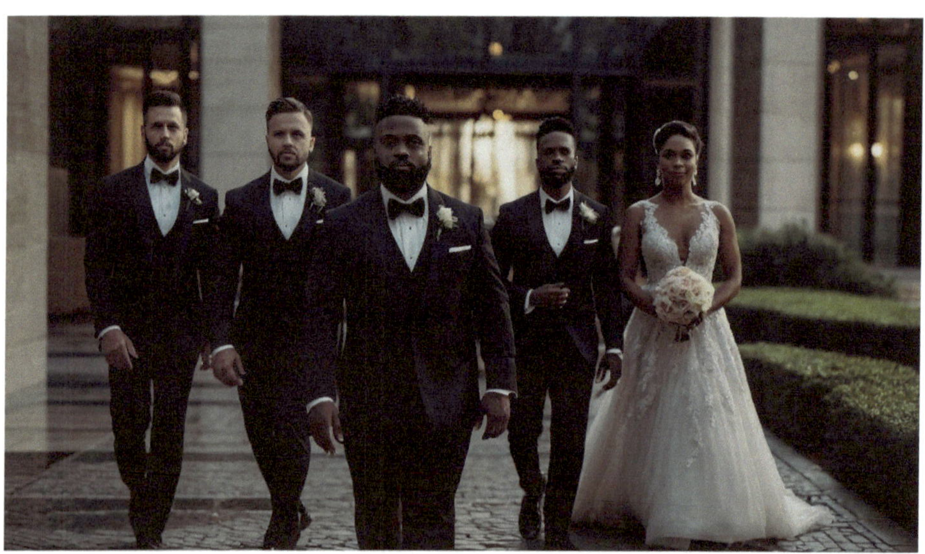

A wedding is one of the best places to show off your style!

- Semi-Formal Wedding Attire: For semi-formal weddings, opt for attire that strikes a balance between formal and casual, such as a tailored blazer paired with dress trousers and a dress shirt, or a lightweight suit in a lighter colour palette such as beige or light grey. Accessories such as a pocket square, a leather belt, and dress shoes add a touch of sophistication to your semi-formal wedding ensemble.

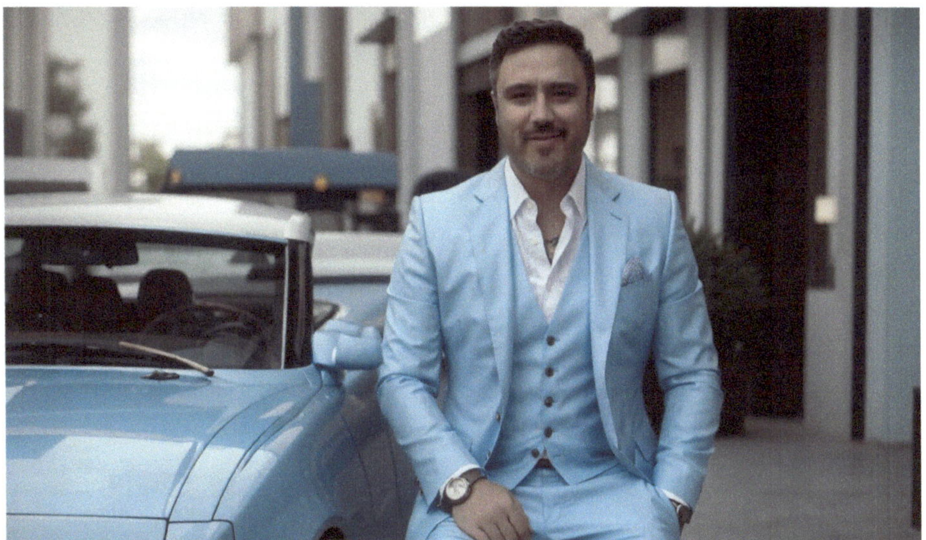

Be daring, you know that you want to!

Dressing for Celebrations and Milestones

Celebrations and milestones are a time for joy and reflection, requiring attire that is celebratory, festive, and appropriate for the occasion. Whether it's a milestone birthday, an anniversary celebration, or a holiday gathering, dressing with style and elegance ensures that you look and feel your best while commemorating life's special moments.

- Cocktail Attire: For cocktail parties and festive gatherings, opt for attire that is sophisticated and stylish, such as a tailored suit in a darker colour palette paired with a dress shirt and a patterned tie, or a sleek blazer paired with dress trousers and a dress shirt. Accessories such as a pocket square, a statement watch, and dress shoes add a touch of elegance to your cocktail attire, ensuring that you stand out for all the right reasons.

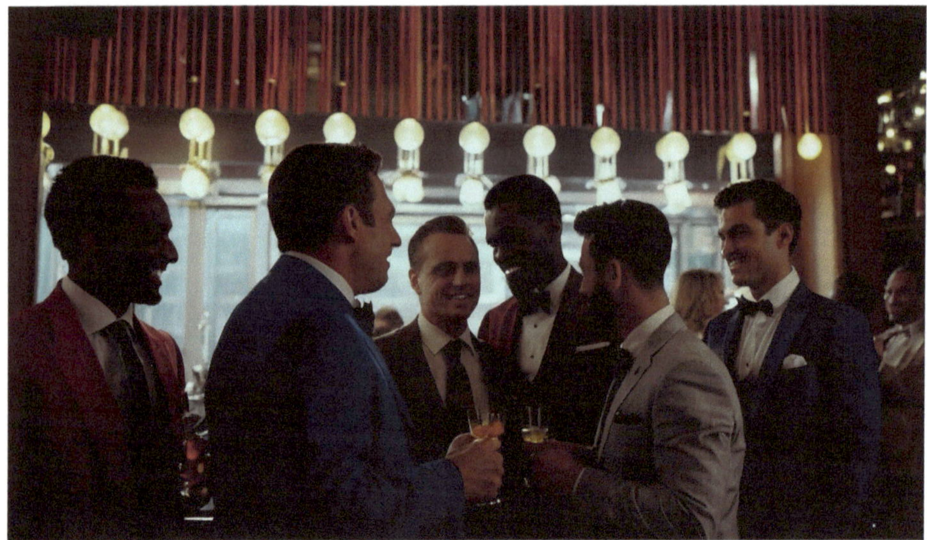

Celebrate in style.

- Festive Attire: For holiday gatherings and festive occasions, opt for attire that is celebratory and colourful, such as a patterned blazer paired with dress trousers and a dress shirt, or a sweater paired with chinos and loafers. Incorporate festive colours and patterns into your ensemble, and accessorise with seasonal accents such as a holiday tie or a statement scarf to add a touch of whimsy and charm to your festive attire.

Funeral Attire: Navigating Cultural Sensitivities

A quick word about funerals. Funerals are a time of mourning and reflection, requiring attire that is respectful and sombre. While black is traditionally worn in Western cultures to symbolise mourning and respect, other cultures, such as in Eastern and

Chinese traditions, may have different colour associations. In Eastern cultures, white is often worn to symbolise mourning and purity, while in Japanese and Western funerals, black or dark colours are typically worn. It's important to be mindful of cultural sensitivities and dress accordingly when attending a funeral, respecting the traditions and customs of the bereaved family.

By mastering the art of formal dressing and navigating dress codes with elegance, you can ensure that you look and feel your best while honouring the significance of life's special moments.

Chapter 7: Icons of Style: Drawing Inspiration from the Masters

In the world of men's fashion, there are those whose sense of style transcends trends and leaves an indelible mark on the fabric of history. From classic Hollywood icons to modern-day influencers, these masters of style serve as beacons of inspiration, guiding us in our quest for sartorial excellence. In this chapter, we delve into the timeless style icons, extract invaluable lessons from their sartorial choices, and explore the art of creating your own signature style.

Timeless Style Icons: From Classic Hollywood to Modern-Day Influencers

Throughout history, certain individuals have captivated the imagination with their impeccable sense of style and effortless elegance. From the debonair charm of classic Hollywood icons to the contemporary influence of modern-day influencers, these timeless style icons continue to inspire and influence the way we dress and present ourselves.

- Classic Hollywood Icons: From the suave sophistication of Cary Grant to the rugged allure of Steve McQueen, classic Hollywood icons epitomise timeless elegance and refined masculinity. Their impeccable tailoring, attention to detail, and understated confidence continue to serve as a source of inspiration for men's fashion aficionados around the world.

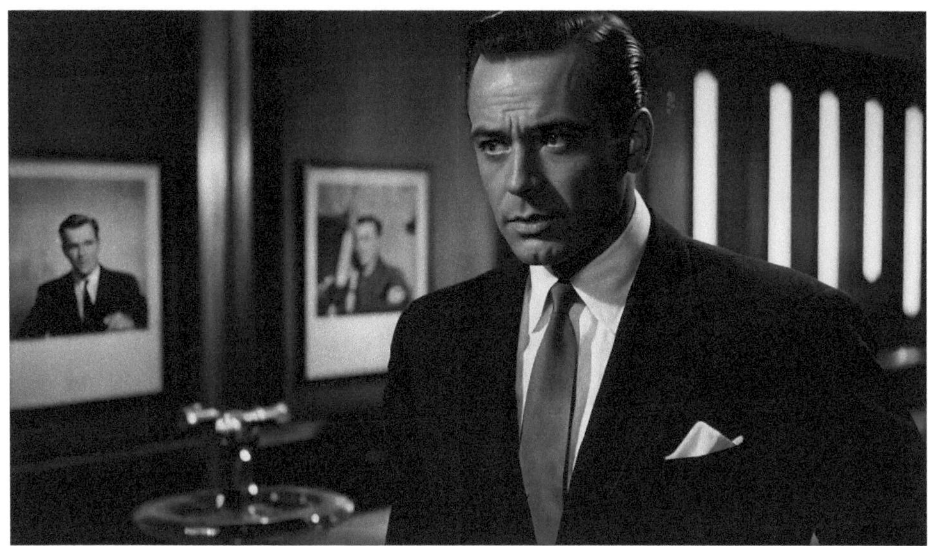

You too can dress like an icon!

- Fashion Mavericks: In the world of modern-day fashion, there are those who push the boundaries of style and challenge convention with their daring sartorial choices. From the avant-garde flair of David Bowie to the eclectic elegance of Pharrell Williams, these fashion mavericks redefine the notion of style and inspire us to embrace our individuality and express ourselves boldly through fashion.

Lessons in Style: What We Can Learn from the Masters

Beyond their impeccable sense of style, the masters of fashion impart invaluable lessons in sartorial elegance, confidence, and self-expression. By studying their sartorial choices and understanding the principles that underpin their iconic looks, we can glean valuable insights into the art of dressing well and presenting ourselves with grace and sophistication.

- Attention to Detail: From the perfect fit of a well-tailored suit to the subtle nuances of accessorising with elegance, attention to detail is paramount in mastering the art of style. By paying attention to the finer details of our attire and grooming, we can elevate our look from ordinary to extraordinary and exude confidence and sophistication in every aspect of our appearance.
- Confidence and Self-Expression: Style is more than just what we wear; it's a reflection of who we are and how we choose to present ourselves to the world. By embracing our individuality and expressing ourselves authentically through fashion, we can exude confidence and charisma that is truly timeless and irresistible.

Creating Your Own Signature Style

While drawing inspiration from the masters of style is invaluable, true sartorial mastery lies in creating your own signature style that is a reflection of your unique personality, tastes, and preferences. By experimenting with different looks, incorporating elements from various style icons, and staying true to yourself, you can develop a signature style that is distinctly yours and exudes confidence, elegance, and sophistication.

- Define Your Aesthetic: Take the time to explore different styles, aesthetics, and influences to determine what resonates with you on a personal level. Whether it's the classic elegance of a tailored suit or the casual cool of streetwear, define your aesthetic and embrace it wholeheartedly as the foundation of your signature style.
- Experiment and Evolve: Style is a journey of self-discovery and self-expression, and it's important to embrace experimentation and evolution in your sartorial journey. Try new looks, experiment with different silhouettes and colour

palettes, and don't be afraid to step out of your comfort zone to discover new facets of your personal style.
- Stay True to Yourself: Above all, stay true to yourself and your unique sense of style. Your signature style should be a reflection of your personality, tastes, and preferences, and it should make you feel confident, empowered, and authentic. Embrace what makes you unique, and let your individuality shine through in every aspect of your wardrobe and presentation.

By drawing inspiration from the masters and staying true to yourself, you can cultivate a style that is truly timeless, authentic, and effortlessly elegant.

Chapter 8: Navigating Trends: Incorporating Contemporary Fashion

In the ever-evolving landscape of men's fashion, navigating trends is a delicate balance between embracing the latest styles and staying true to timeless elegance. In this chapter, we explore the art of incorporating contemporary fashion into your wardrobe, striking a harmonious balance between modern trends and timeless pieces, and knowing when to embrace or avoid fleeting fads.

Incorporating Trends with Timeless Pieces

Integrating contemporary fashion trends into your wardrobe allows you to infuse freshness and relevance into your style while still maintaining a foundation of timeless pieces that withstand the test of time. By strategically incorporating trends into your wardrobe, you can create dynamic and versatile looks that are both fashionable and enduring.

- Key Trend Pieces: Identify key trend pieces that resonate with your personal style and complement your existing wardrobe. Whether it's a statement outerwear piece, a bold patterned shirt, or a pair of on-trend sneakers, choose trend pieces that add interest and personality to your ensemble while still maintaining a cohesive aesthetic.
- Mix and Match: Mix contemporary trend pieces with timeless wardrobe staples to create balanced and stylish outfits. Pair trend pieces with classic basics such as tailored trousers, a crisp white shirt, or a well-fitted blazer to create a polished and sophisticated look that seamlessly blends modern trends with timeless elegance.

The Art of Balance: Mixing Classic and Contemporary Styles

The art of incorporating contemporary fashion lies in striking a harmonious balance between classic and contemporary styles. By blending classic wardrobe staples with modern trend pieces, you can create looks that are both stylish and timeless, exuding confidence and sophistication.

- Classic Wardrobe Staples: Invest in classic wardrobe staples such as tailored suits, crisp white shirts, and well-fitted denim jeans that serve as the foundation of your wardrobe. These timeless pieces provide a versatile canvas for incorporating contemporary trends and can be styled in endless combinations for a variety of occasions.
- Contemporary Trend Pieces: Experiment with contemporary trend pieces such as statement outerwear, bold patterns, and unconventional accessories to add a modern edge to your ensemble. Choose trend pieces that complement your personal style and enhance your overall aesthetic, and incorporate them strategically into your wardrobe for a fresh and dynamic look.

Knowing When to Embrace or Avoid Trends

While incorporating contemporary fashion trends into your wardrobe can add excitement and relevance to your style, it's important to know when to embrace or avoid fleeting fads. By understanding your personal style preferences, lifestyle needs, and the longevity of a trend, you can make informed decisions about which trends to incorporate into your wardrobe and which to avoid.

- Personal Style Preferences: Consider your personal style preferences and how a trend aligns with your aesthetic and wardrobe needs. Choose trends that resonate with your individual style and enhance your overall look, and avoid trends that feel forced or incongruent with your personal aesthetic.

- Lifestyle Needs: Take into account your lifestyle needs and the practicality of a trend in your day-to-day life. Choose trends that fit seamlessly into your lifestyle and complement your daily activities, and avoid trends that are impractical or uncomfortable for your everyday routine.
- Longevity of a Trend: Evaluate the longevity of a trend and consider whether it has staying power beyond the current season. Choose trends that have lasting appeal and can be incorporated into your wardrobe for seasons to come, and avoid trends that are overly fleeting or likely to go out of style quickly.

In this chapter, we have explored the art of incorporating contemporary fashion into your wardrobe, striking a harmonious balance between modern trends and timeless pieces, and knowing when to embrace or avoid fleeting fads. By strategically incorporating trends with timeless pieces and understanding your personal style preferences, lifestyle needs, and the longevity of a trend, you can navigate the ever-changing landscape of men's fashion with confidence and style.

Chapter 9: Elevating Your Look with Accessories

Accessories are the finishing touches that add flair and personality to your ensemble, allowing you to express your individual style and elevate your look with finesse. From classic essentials to statement pieces, mastering the art of accessorising is key to creating polished and sophisticated outfits.

- Classic Essentials: Invest in classic accessories that serve as timeless staples in your wardrobe, such as a quality leather belt, a versatile watch, and a pair of stylish sunglasses. These classic essentials complement a variety of outfits and add a touch of refinement to your ensemble.

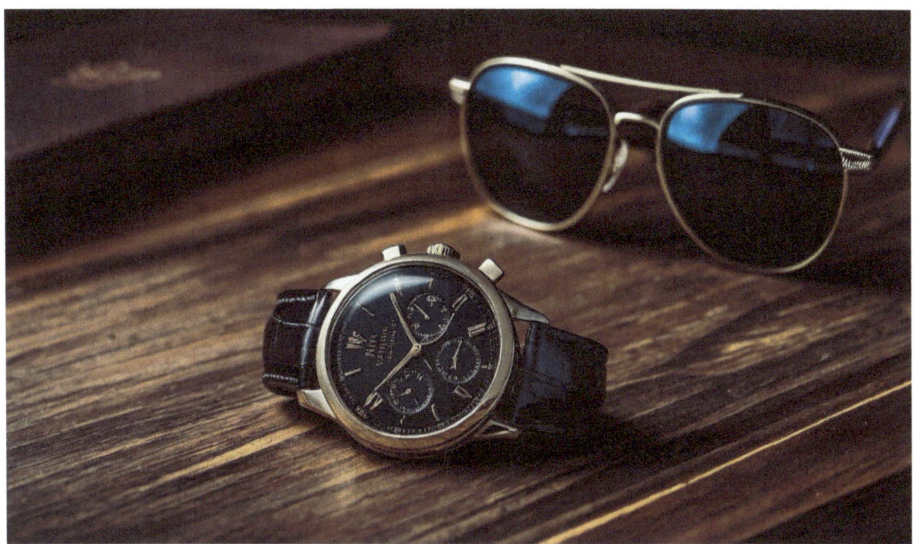

- Statement Pieces: Experiment with statement accessories that make a bold statement and add personality to your look, such as a patterned tie, a vibrant pocket square, or a statement watch. Choose statement pieces that reflect your personal style and add visual interest to your outfit without overwhelming the overall aesthetic.

The Gentleman's Guide to Grooming

Grooming is an essential component of presenting yourself with confidence and sophistication. From skincare to haircare, mastering the gentleman's guide to grooming ensures that you look and feel your best, exuding confidence and elegance in every aspect of your appearance.

- Skincare Routine: Establish a skincare routine that addresses your specific skin concerns and maintains a healthy and youthful complexion. Cleanse, exfoliate, moisturise, and protect your skin with quality skincare products that are suited to your skin type and needs.
- Hair Care Regimen: Maintain a well-groomed appearance with a hair care regimen that keeps your hair looking healthy and stylish. Regularly shampoo, condition, and style your hair with quality hair care products that enhance its natural texture and shine.

Maintaining Your Wardrobe: Care and Storage Tips

Proper care and maintenance are essential for preserving the longevity and quality of your wardrobe. From laundering to storing, mastering care and storage tips ensures that your garments remain in pristine condition, ready to be worn with confidence and style.

- Laundering: Follow care instructions on garment labels and launder your clothing with care to avoid damage and preserve their quality. Sort clothing by colour and fabric, use appropriate detergents and washing temperatures, and air-dry or tumble-dry garments as recommended to maintain their shape and colour.

- Storage: Store your clothing properly to prevent wrinkles, creases, and damage. Invest in quality hangers, garment bags, and storage containers to protect your clothing from dust, moths, and other environmental factors. Fold knitwear, hang shirts and jackets, and store suits and coats in breathable garment bags to maintain their shape and freshness.

By paying attention to the finishing touches, from classic accessories to grooming rituals and wardrobe maintenance, you can elevate your look with sophistication and style, ensuring that you always look and feel your best.

Chapter 10: Beyond Fashion: Cultivating Confidence and Presence

Fashion is more than just the clothes we wear; it's a powerful tool for cultivating confidence, self-expression, and presence in the world. In this final chapter, we explore the psychology of dressing well, the transformative power of fashion in building confidence and self-expression, and the timeless allure of embracing style as a lifestyle choice that transcends trends.

The Psychology of Dressing Well

The clothes we wear have a profound impact on how we perceive ourselves and how others perceive us. The psychology of dressing well is rooted in the concept of "enclothed cognition," which suggests that the clothes we wear can influence our thoughts, feelings, and behaviour.

- Self-Perception: Dressing well can boost our self-perception and self-esteem, instilling a sense of confidence, competence, and empowerment. When we dress in clothing that makes us feel good about ourselves, we are more likely to project a positive self-image and exude confidence in our interactions with others.

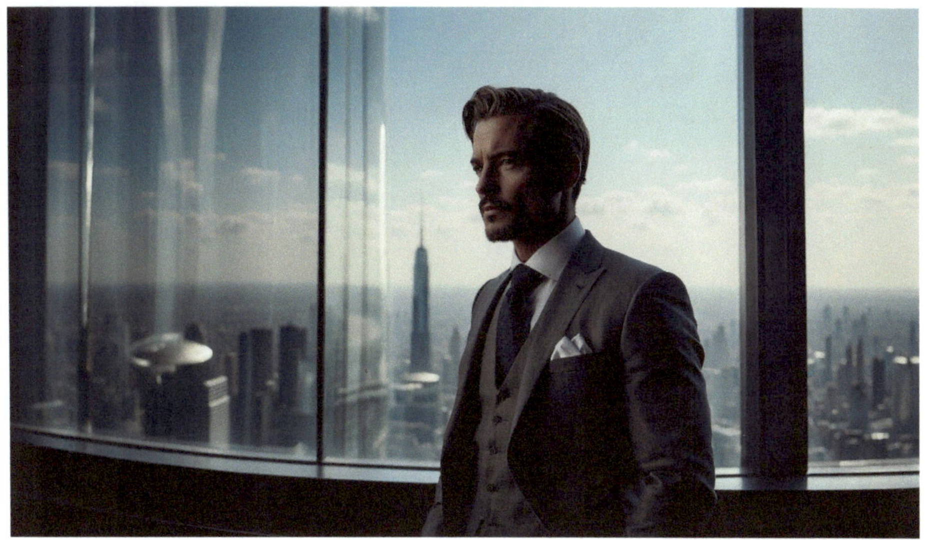

The future is yours.

- Social Perception: Dressing well also influences how others perceive us, shaping their initial impressions and judgments. When we present ourselves with care and attention to detail, we signal to others that we are competent, trustworthy, and worthy of respect, enhancing our social standing and influencing how others interact with us.

Confidence and Self-Expression through Fashion

Fashion is a form of self-expression, allowing us to communicate our personality, values, and identity to the world. By embracing fashion as a means of self-expression, we can cultivate confidence, assert our individuality, and create a lasting impression.

- Authenticity: Dressing in a way that reflects our authentic self allows us to express our true identity and values, fostering a sense of confidence and self-assurance. By embracing our unique style preferences and wearing clothing that resonates with who we are, we can project authenticity and integrity in our personal and professional lives.

- Creativity: Fashion is a creative outlet that allows us to experiment with different styles, colours, and silhouettes, expressing our creativity and individuality in the way we dress. By embracing fashion as a form of creative expression, we can tap into our innate creativity, explore new possibilities, and develop our personal style with confidence and flair.

Embracing Timeless Style as a Lifestyle Choice

Beyond fleeting trends and seasonal fads, timeless style offers a timeless allure that transcends the whims of fashion. Embracing timeless style as a lifestyle choice allows us to cultivate a wardrobe that is classic, versatile, and enduring, reflecting our commitment to quality, craftsmanship, and timeless elegance.

- Quality over Quantity: Embrace quality over quantity when building your wardrobe, investing in timeless pieces that are well-made, versatile, and built to last. By prioritising quality craftsmanship and timeless design, you can curate a wardrobe that stands the test of time and reflects your commitment to enduring style.
- Mindful Consumption: Practise mindful consumption by making thoughtful and intentional choices about the clothing and accessories you purchase. Consider the environmental and social impact of your fashion choices, support sustainable and ethical brands, and prioritise investment pieces that bring value and joy to your wardrobe.

By understanding the psychology of dressing well, embracing fashion as a form of self-expression, and embracing timeless style as a lifestyle choice, you can harness the transformative power of fashion to project confidence, authenticity, and timeless elegance in every aspect of your life. Anyone can learn and apply these principles and bring about a change in their outward appearance and more besides.

Conclusion: Embracing Your Personal Journey in Timeless Style

As we conclude our exploration into the realm of timeless style, it's important to remember that fashion is not just about the clothes we wear; it's about the journey of self-discovery, self-expression, and personal growth that unfolds with each outfit we choose. Embracing timeless style is not about adhering to rigid rules or following fleeting trends; it's about cultivating a sense of confidence, authenticity, and presence that radiates from within.

As you embark on your personal journey in timeless style, I encourage you to go out and apply the tips and insights shared in this book. Experiment with different styles, silhouettes, and colours to discover what resonates with you on a personal level. Become a student of style, finding inspiration in sources like fashion magazines, old movies, and the world around you. Pay attention to the way clothing makes you feel and how it influences your thoughts, feelings, and behaviour. Allow yourself the freedom to express your unique personality and individuality through your fashion choices, knowing that true style is a reflection of who you are and what you stand for.

Remember that timeless style is not about perfection; it's about embracing the journey of self-discovery and self-expression with grace and confidence. Be open to trying new things, stepping out of your comfort zone, and embracing the unexpected twists and turns that come with personal style. Trust your instincts, listen to your inner voice, and have the courage to forge your own path in the world of fashion.

As you navigate the exciting and ever-changing landscape of timeless style, remember that the most important accessory you can wear is confidence. Stand tall, walk with purpose, and embrace your unique sense of style with pride and conviction.

Whether you're dressed in a tailored suit or a casual ensemble, let your confidence and authenticity shine through, knowing that true style comes from within.

The world is your runway, and your personal style is your unique expression of self. Embrace it, own it, and let it inspire you to live your best life with confidence, authenticity, and timeless elegance.